The Bible Promises of Healing

16 Letters for Mom

By

Ivan Thompson

Table of Contents

Preface

God has blessed me with three moms: My natural mom, Walterine, who is alive and well; my dad's current wife, Valerie; and my mom, "Earnestine." I am truly blessed!

This is a book written for my Mom, Earnstine. Though the Holy Spirit told me to write this book for my mom, Earnestine, I knew that He had a higher purpose and a broader audience that was supposed to benefit from it.

In this book, I will often address my mom and talk as though I am talking to her. Please don't let that keep you from benefiting from the Bible truths in the book. I'm speaking to my mom out of love for her and, more importantly, out of the love God has for her.

Since God has the same love for you, it's more than okay to imagine that it is God speaking to you out of His great love for you.

I urge you to share this book with anyone who is battling sickness and disease, especially terminal illness. Money should not be an obstacle. I would gladly make a transcript of this book available to any who feels that they need it but can't afford it. Contact me at ivan.arizona@yahoo.com.

God bless you as you read this book!

Dedication (How This Book Came About)

On the 30th of December 2017, I woke up and while I was lying in bed praying for you, the Holy Spirit started ministering to me the idea of writing you a series of letters on healing. As I was lying in bed praying Holy Spirit just started walking me through so many of the significant elements of healing that I have learned from Kenneth and Gloria Copeland, Keith Moore, Apostle Fred Price, and directly from scripture as I have studied the subject of healing.

I have watched so much suffering in your family over the years. I have watched you serve and minister to the sick members of your family. The enemy has mounted his attack now with increasing focus on you. I believe this is why the Holy Spirit inspired me to write these letters for you and gave me an urgency to get them to you.

Isaiah 59:19 (NKJV) says, "When the enemy comes in like a flood, The Spirit of the LORD will lift up a standard against him." The enemy has come in like a flood in your life, attacking your body in multiple places, and now the Spirit of the Lord, the Holy Spirit, is raising up a standard, a banner, a flag, with the Words of God written upon it. Your ailments are not merely the result of old age or heredity. They are not your fault or a punishment for a former sin. Most importantly, they are not the will of God for your life, nor are they part of God's testing of your faith or love for Him.

The standard that the Lord will raise in these letters is that God loves you. He loves you more than I ever could, more than you could ever understand or imagine. He loved you so much that He sent His Son to give His life for you. He loved you so much that He sent angels to watch over you. He loved you so much that He sent the Holy Spirit to guide you and minister to you and help you daily. He loves you so much that He sent His word to heal you.

Prayerfully read these letters and receive your healing! Love you, mom!

Why Did Jesus Come?

1 John 4:9 (NKJV): "In this the love of God was manifested toward us, that God has sent His only begotten Son into the world, that we might live through Him."

1 John 3:8 (NKJV): "…For this purpose the Son of God was manifested, that He might destroy the works of the devil."

Acts 10:38 (NLT): "And you know that God anointed Jesus of Nazareth with the Holy Spirit and with power. Then Jesus went around doing good and healing all who were oppressed by the devil, for God was with him."

Luke 11:14-15, 18-20 (NKJV): "And He was casting out a demon, and it was mute. So it was, when the demon had gone out, that the mute spoke; and the multitudes marveled. But some of them said, He casts out demons by Beelzebub, the ruler of the demons. If Satan also is divided against himself, how will his kingdom stand? Because you say I cast out demons by Beelzebub. And if I cast out demons by Beelzebub, by whom do your sons cast them out? Therefore they will be your judges. But if I cast out demons with the finger of God, surely the kingdom of God has come upon you."

It's so easy to think about Jesus coming to earth to seek and save the lost. However, we get so caught up with Jesus being the only way to the Father and eternal life that we forget that He also came to heal. I John 3:8 says that

Jesus came "to destroy the works of the devil." Part of the devil's work was to eternally separate men from the Father. We know that Jesus destroyed that work at the resurrection.

But there were other works that Jesus was sent here to destroy. Acts 10:38 makes it very clear what these works were: "healing all who were oppressed of the devil." So, wherever the devil had made people sick or oppressed them spiritually, Jesus healed them.

Why did Jesus heal? That was part of His assignment. Sickness and disease are works of the devil, and Jesus was sent here to destroy everything that the devil put in place after Adam's fall. Jesus was sent to restore God's original vision for man.

You may have heard the "good news" of the gospel that Jesus came so that your sins could be forgiven and that you could have eternal life. That's good news, but there is more good news.

What is that news? That you don't have to be sick. The same Jesus that came to bring you salvation came to bring you healing. It doesn't matter what caused you to be sick or what disease you have. All sickness has the same remedy; the healing power of God through Jesus Christ.

After World War II, some Japanese soldiers had not received news that war was over and were still trying to fight. When slavery ended in the United States, there were many negro slaves that did not get the good news that they were now ex-slaves.

Many people have never heard the good news that the same Jesus that was sent on assignment to destroy the power of sin was also sent to destroy the power of sickness and every other work of the devil. Receive the good news today. Set your heart to enjoy every benefit that God planned for you when He, in His great mercy, sent His Son to earth for us.

He Healed Them All

Matthew 12:15 (NKJV): "But when Jesus knew it, He withdrew from there. And great multitudes followed Him, and He healed them all."

Luke 6:17-19 (NKJV): "And He came down with them and stood on a level place with a crowd of His disciples and a great multitude of people from all Judea and Jerusalem, and from the seacoast of Tyre and Sidon, who came to hear Him and be healed of their diseases. As well as those who were tormented with unclean spirits. And they were healed. And the whole multitude sought to touch Him, for power went out from Him and healed them all."

Matthew 4:24 (NKJV): "Then His fame went throughout all Syria; and they brought to Him all sick people who were afflicted with various diseases and torments, and those who were demon-possessed, epileptics, and paralytics; and He healed them."

Luke 4:40 (NKJV): "When the sun was setting, all those who had any that were sick with various diseases brought them to Him; and He laid His hands on every one of them and healed them."

Mom, this is one of the most critical yet overlooked teachings of the Bible as it pertains to healing. In these Scriptures, multitudes of people showed up with "various diseases," even people that were paralyzed, and Jesus "healed them all," "every one of them."

There are popular but wrong teachings that some people don't get healed because it was God's will that they stay sick to learn a lesson, to grow spiritually, or because God meant to use that sickness to call that person back to Heaven.

It has always amazed me that this false teaching could prosper for so long against the truth of the Scripture. I used to imagine the multitudes of people as described in the Bible, coming to Jesus for healing and Him telling some of them no. I used to imagine Jesus telling selected people, "oh, this sickness was meant to teach you humility or some other lesson, so you have to keep it; now, please step aside." I had to imagine it because it's so ridiculous that it can't be found anywhere in Scripture.

I know that some people will jump to the "thorn in the flesh" and will touch briefly on that later. But for now, let's just say that if God were trying to teach us the lesson that not everyone gets their healing, wouldn't He put more than one example in the New Testament? Further, if multitudes, everyone, all the people that Jesus laid hands on or prayed for, got healed, why would you choose to identify yourself as one in the "thorn group" who didn't?

It doesn't make sense. This healing-is-not-for-everyone teaching flies in the face of the love of God, the character, and nature of God. It doesn't make sense because it's not true. But men who couldn't explain why a person didn't get healed have chosen to make God less powerful, pull Him down to the level of their personal experience, and blame Him instead of saying, "I don't know why sister so-and-so died after we prayed."

2 Timothy 3:16 (NKJV) says, "All Scripture is given by inspiration of God, and is profitable for doctrine, for reproof, for correction, for instruction in righteousness…" Therefore, we always base our doctrine, our set of beliefs, on the Word of God, not our own experience. If the Bible says that Jesus healed them all, we extend our faith towards that possibility versus our personal experience of people who didn't get healed. **2 Corinthians 5:7 (NKJV)** says, "For we walk by faith, not by sight."

In other letters, you will find more Scriptures that describe the things that must be present for healing to take place. It's almost impossible unless you were the person that didn't get healed to say if all the things were in place for healing to be received. It's hard to say that if something was done differently that a loved one might have gotten healed. But does that justify saying that the power of God has somehow lessened 2000+ years later?

It is so much better to say, in humility, that I don't know why some people didn't get their healing, but I believe that I will be part of the "all," "the multitude," "the everyone" that will.

Go to the Doctor/Take Your Medicine

Proverbs 8:12 (KJV): "I wisdom dwell with prudence, and find out knowledge of witty inventions."

Proverbs 8:12 (WEB): "I wisdom dwell with prudence, and find out knowledge of ingenious inventions."

Because most of these letters will deal with receiving your healing by faith, it might seem that I am against doctors or medicines or surgery. Quite the contrary. The Bible says that God gives us "the knowledge of witty inventions." I believe that God has always been at work on the earth, giving scientists clues and aid to defeat sickness and disease.

I used to believe that all the Old Testament laws that God gave the children of Israel about things that should be treated as unclean were given to protect them from disease. They had laws governing what happened if you touched a dead body or touched someone who was sick, etc. I believed that God was protecting them long before microscopes, bacteria, and germs were discovered.

Today I researched this theory and found out it was true! I found many articles that showed how the Old Testament laws governing what was unclean helped keep the children of Israel healthy and safe from diseases:

"Biblical admonitions also include avoiding contact with animals that have died or with whatever has touched them (see Leviticus 11:32–40). Porous earthen vessels, potentially contaminated, were to be destroyed to avoid spreading disease. These biblical regulations are consistent with sound microbiological techniques, and are fundamentally important in fighting infectious disease. It was the priests' job to teach and explain these laws. Priests were to designate as unclean those who had contagious diseases characterized by skin rashes, such as leprosy, measles, smallpox and scarlet fever. Such individuals were to be isolated from others to prevent the spread of disease (see Leviticus 13). These biblical guidelines are the basis of medically sound quarantine procedures that have been used for centuries. Bible guidelines include avoiding contact with personal items of sick people that could transmit germs (Leviticus 13:47–59). Contaminated items were to be washed or burned (which destroys microorganisms). Biblical health instructions even applied to dwellings—mold or fungal growth had to be scraped off, or a house would be quarantined or demolished. Cracks, which harbor ticks and other disease-bearing bugs, were to be plastered (Leviticus 14:33–48). The priest functioned as both a public health educator and a building inspector, to promote health and prevent disease.

The Bible acknowledges that body fluids can be a vehicle for transmitting disease (Leviticus 15). Contact with human waste materials, nasal discharges, tears, saliva and other fluids, or contact with soiled towels or linen, can spread infectious disease. Trachoma—a leading cause of blindness—is spread by contact with soiled hand towels and eye-seeking flies. Those coming into contact with fluids from a sick person had to wash their hands and clothes in water, bathe, and remain isolated from other people until evening as a precaution against spreading disease (Leviticus 15:11). Men and women were to bathe after having sexual relations (Leviticus 15:18). The purpose of these sanitary laws was to promote health and prevent disease (Leviticus 15:31). They were not just ceremonial rituals.

One of the most practical and powerful biblical admonitions states that when people dwell together, human wastes are to be deposited outside the living area and buried (Deuteronomy 23:12–14). This prevents waste materials from coming in contact with people, flies and other organisms that transmit disease. It also prevents the contamination of water supplies. Many diseases, such as diarrhea, dysentery, hookworm, roundworms, cholera and typhoid, result from contact with human waste."

(Winnail, 2002)

Long before the discovery of diseases, God was helping the children of Israel "find out knowledge of" helpful medical practices. If God went through so much trouble to help keep them from being sick back, then would He do less to protect us now, as believers in Jesus Christ?

I believe that God can work through a doctor, surgeon, dietician, pharmacist, etc. I do believe that you should pray for them as they devise their treatment plan for you. I believe that you should pray for the advice they give you, and unless you have a solid track record of healing by faith, you probably should follow their advice.

What do I mean by track record? Years ago, Dr. Frederick K.C. Price preached a sermon about your "faith photo album." He said in your faith photo album are things that you can point to and say God did that for me, and He helped me here and delivered me there.

In my faith photo album, I have many healing testimonies. I have laid hands on myself and my children and seen fevers broken. My back was broken in 1983, and I was in great pain most of the time. I was supernaturally healed to the point that I could lift weights, run, play competitive basketball and football, etc. without pain up to this very day in 2017.

I have been supernaturally healed of Irritable Bowel Syndrome (IBS) and Gastroesophageal Reflux Disease (GERD)—no more need for medications. I was supernaturally healed of several sports injuries without surgery (surgery was prescribed but not needed), a sports hernia, a severe knee injury, and a severe injury to my ankle/foot.

Each healing helped build my faith for the next healing. That's not everybody's testimony. There is no condemnation if it's not. There have been many other things for which I have gone to the doctor or have taken medicine. My faith victories merely mean that most of the time, I look to my faith as the source of my healing, and I prayerfully consider what the doctor prescribes. I praise God for doctors who have helped me get better or identified the area where I need to focus my faith.

I believe that God is going to heal you. I believe it is His will for your life. These letters were meant to help build your faith. Believing that God can use doctors and medication can most definitely be a big part of that. And for everything that the doctors can't do and medicines can't do, God Himself is undoubtedly capable, willing, and available to.

God's Motivation is Always Love

John 3:16 (ESV): "For God so loved the world, that he gave his only Son, that whoever believes in him should not perish but have eternal life."

Romans 8:32 (NKJV): "He who did not spare His own Son, but delivered Him up for us all, how shall He not with Him also freely give us all things?"

Ephesians 3:14-19 (NKJV): "For this reason I bow my knees to the Father of our Lord Jesus Christ, from whom the whole family in heaven and earth is named, that He would grant you, according to the riches of His glory, to be strengthened with might through His Spirit in the inner man, may be able to comprehend with all the saints what is the width and length and depth and height—to know the love of Christ which passes knowledge; that you may be filled with all the fullness of God."

1 John 4:16, 18-19 (NKJV): "And we have known and believed the love that God has for us. God is love, and he who abides in love abides in God, and God in him. There is no fear in love; but perfect love casts out fear, because fear involves torment. But he who fears has not been made perfect in love. We love Him because He first loved us."

1 John 3:1 (NKJV): "Behold what manner of love the Father has bestowed on us, that we should be called children of God..."

Romans 5:5 (NKJV): "Now hope does not disappoint, because the love of God has been poured out in our hearts by the Holy Spirit who was given to us."

Romans 5:5 (NLT): "And this hope will not lead to disappointment. For we know how dearly God loves us, because he has given us the Holy Spirit to fill our hearts with his love."

Luke 11:13 (NKJV): "If you then, being evil, know how to give good gifts to your children, how much more will your heavenly Father give the Holy Spirit to those who ask Him!"

Matthew 7:11 (NKJV): "Ask, and it will be given to you; seek, and you will find; knock, and it will be opened to you. For everyone who asks receives, and he who seeks finds, and to him who knocks it will be opened. Or what man is there among you who, if his son asks for bread, will give him a stone? Or if he asks for a fish, will he give him a serpent? If you then, being evil, know how to give good gifts to your children, how much more will your Father who is in heaven give good things to those who ask Him!"

Mom, what should jump out at you in the Scriptures is that God loves us so much. He loved us so much that He sent His only Son, Jesus, to restore the relationship, the intimate fellowship that He enjoyed with Adam and Eve in the garden before the fall. Romans 8:32

above basically says if He would give us Jesus, why wouldn't He "freely give" us anything else we need.

We have been taught so many wrong things about God. So many people, in their misunderstanding of God, especially the God of the Old Testament, try to make God schizophrenic. Meaning that one moment, He is loving us, and the next minute He's destroying us.

The quote from Ephesians chapter 3 tells us that we need the help of the Holy Spirit working within us to be able to grasp and understand "the width, length, and depth" of God's love for us. This verse says that God's love for us is a love that surpasses knowledge. That means we can't even begin to understand God's love for us with our natural minds; we need the help of the Holy Spirit.

I pray that the Holy Spirit helps you even now "to know and believe the love God has for you." (1 John 4:16). That as you supernaturally come to know this love, this perfect love, that it would cast out any fear/terror of God that might exist in your heart. I pray that you would understand that we love God because He first loved us. His love is the love that "has been poured into our hearts by the Holy Spirit. Out of that love, God has called us His "children."

As the revelation of the love of God in these Scriptures grows in your heart, it will affect your ideas about God. You're a good mom, but Matt 7:11 says that any parent we can think of is relatively evil in comparison to God. I could say it like this: any parent on their best day could never be the parent that God is to us.

Matt 7:11 goes on to say, "If you then, being evil, know how to give good gifts to your children, how much more will your Father who is in heaven give good things to those who ask Him!" If you ask God for healing, He won't give you suffering or death. That is a perverted understanding of God that comes straight from the devil!

Satan first told the angels in heaven that God didn't have their best interests in mind and that they'd be better off following him, one-third believed him and lost everything. Next, he told Adam and Eve that God wasn't good and that He wasn't loving because He was keeping something from them. He told them that listening to him was better, and they could eat from the tree. They did and lost everything.

Don't listen to Satan or the echoes of his voice that may come even from well-meaning people as they try to tell you that God is not loving or the giver of good things. If you ask God for good things, He will give you good things.

Our Father in Heaven is the giver of good things. Healing is a good thing. Walking in health is a good thing. Pray for these good things and believe that a good God gives good things! Amen.

Salvation and Healing Received the Same Way

Ephesians 2:8-9 (ESV): "For by grace you have been saved through faith. And this is not your own doing; it is the gift of God, not a result of works, so that no one may boast."

Romans 10:9-10 (NKJV): "That if you confess with your mouth the Lord Jesus and believe in your heart that God has raised Him from the dead, you will be saved. For with the heart one believes unto righteousness, and with the mouth confession is made unto salvation. For the Scripture says, Whoever believes on Him will not be put to shame. For there is no distinction between Jew and Greek, for the same Lord over all is rich to all who call upon Him.
For whoever calls on the name of the LORD shall be saved. How then shall they call on Him in whom they have not believed? And how shall they believe in Him of whom they have not heard? And how shall they hear without a preacher?"

Romans 10:17 (NKJV): "So then faith comes by hearing, and hearing by the word of God."

Mom, you have heard Ephesians 2:8-9 many times over the years that grace saves us through faith, not by any works that we could do. Further, when you accepted Christ, you did so by believing in your heart that God raised Jesus from the dead and confessing it with your mouth. Romans 10:10 says the belief in Jesus' death, burial, and resurrection and your confession of that belief made you righteous or put you in right standing with God eternally.

How did you get the faith to believe that Christ died on the cross for our sins? You heard it. You heard it preached, or you may have read it in the Bible. The chances are that you have heard it repeatedly. It is one of the things that is preached in most Christian churches every Sunday at an altar call or close of the service. However you heard it, the faith to believe it came by hearing it and then believing it and confessing it. You are not in heaven now, but you have salvation just as undoubtedly as you have air. You know, that you know that you are saved, that you have salvation. Again, because you have heard the Word of God in that area over and over, and it built your faith.

What if you heard the Scriptures over and over about how Jesus healed in the Bible? If you heard those words over and over, it would build your faith because faith for healing comes the same way faith for salvation comes. It comes by hearing and hearing the Word of God. You have to hear scriptures on healing to build your faith to be healed.

Once you build your faith for healing, then by faith, you begin to believe in your heart that you receive healing, and you confess with your mouth that you receive healing. Just like believing salvation Scriptures leads to righteousness, believing healing Scriptures leads to healing. Just like confession is a demonstration of your faith that you received your salvation, confession is a demonstration of your faith that you received your healing.

But what if you don't hear healing Scriptures in your church? Then you need to hear it somewhere else. Put on a CD, a television, or internet broadcast, or read the Scriptures in this book out loud. Faith can come by hearing the Word of God when you read it aloud.

In the letters that follow, I will give you many, many Scriptures that you can read and say aloud to build your faith and receive your healing.

According to Your Faith

Matthew 9:28-29 (NKJV): "And when He had come into the house, the blind men came to Him. And Jesus said to them, Do you believe that I am able to do this? They said to Him, Yes, Lord. Then He touched their eyes, saying, According to your faith let it be to you."

Matthew 9:20-22 (KJV): "And, behold, a woman, which was diseased with an issue of blood twelve years, came behind him, and touched the hem of his garment: For she said within herself, If I may but touch his garment, I shall be whole. But Jesus turned him about, and when he saw her, he said, Daughter, be of good comfort; thy faith hath made thee whole. And the woman was made whole from that hour."

Matthew 8:5-10 (KJV): "And when Jesus was entered into Capernaum, there came unto him a centurion, beseeching him, And saying, Lord, my servant lieth at home sick of the palsy, grievously tormented. And Jesus saith unto him, I will come and heal him. The centurion answered and said, Lord, I am not worthy that thou shouldest come under my roof: but speak the word only, and my servant shall be healed. For I am a man under authority, having soldiers under me: and I say to this man, Go, and he goeth; and to another, Come, and he cometh; and to my servant, Do this, and he doeth it. When Jesus heard it, he marvelled, and said to them that followed, Verily I say unto you, I have not found so great faith, no, not in Israel."

Luke 8:41-42, 49-55 (KJV): "And, behold, there came a man named Jairus, and he was a ruler of the synagogue:

and he fell down at Jesus' feet, and besought him that he would come into his house: For he had one only daughter, about twelve years of age, and she lay a dying. But as he went the people thronged him…While he yet spake, there cometh one from the ruler of the synagogue's house, saying to him, Thy daughter is dead; trouble not the Master. But when Jesus heard it, he answered him, saying, Fear not: believe only, and she shall be made whole. And when he came into the house, he suffered no man to go in, save Peter, and James, and John, and the father and the mother of the maiden. And all wept, and bewailed her: but he said, Weep not; she is not dead, but sleepeth. And they laughed him to scorn, knowing that she was dead. And he put them all out, and took her by the hand, and called, saying, Maid, arise. And her spirit came again, and she arose straightway: and he commanded to give her meat."

Mark 9:17-29 (NKJV): "Then one of the crowd answered and said, Teacher, I brought You my son, who has a mute spirit. And wherever it seizes him, it throws him down; he foams at the mouth, gnashes his teeth, and becomes rigid. So I spoke to Your disciples, that they should cast it out, but they could not. He answered him and said, O faithless generation, how long shall I be with you? How long shall I bear with you? Bring him to Me. Then they brought him to Him. And when he saw Him, immediately the spirit convulsed him, and he fell on the ground and wallowed, foaming at the mouth. So He asked his father, how long has this been happening to him? And he said, from childhood. And often he has thrown him both into the fire and into the water to destroy him. But if You can do anything, have compassion on us and help us. Jesus said to him, If you can believe, all things are possible to him who believes. Jesus said to him, If you can believe, all things are possible to him who believes. When Jesus saw that the people came running together, He rebuked the unclean spirit, saying to it: Deaf and dumb spirit, I command you, come out of him and enter him no more! Then the spirit cried out, convulsed him greatly, and came out of him. And he became as one dead, so that many said, He is dead. But Jesus took him by the hand and lifted him up, and he arose. And when He had come into the house, His disciples asked Him privately, Why could we not cast it out? So He said to them, This kind can come out by nothing but prayer and fasting.”

Matthew 15:21-28 (NKJV): “And behold, a woman of Canaan came from that region and cried out to Him, saying, Have mercy on me, O Lord, Son of David! My daughter is severely demon-possessed. But He answered her not a word. And His disciples came and urged Him, saying, Send her away, for she cries out after us. But He answered and said, I was not sent except to the lost sheep of the house of Israel. Then she came and worshiped Him, saying, Lord, help me! But He answered and said, It is not good to take the children’s bread and throw it to the little dogs. And she said, Yes, Lord, yet even the little dogs eat the crumbs which fall from their masters’ table. Then Jesus answered and said to her, O woman, great is your faith!

Let it be to you as you desire. And her daughter was healed from that very hour."

Acts 3:2, 16 (NKJV): "And a certain man lame from his mother's womb was carried, whom they laid daily at the gate of the temple which is called Beautiful, to ask alms from those who entered the temple; who, seeing Peter and John about to go into the temple, asked for alms. And fixing his eyes on him, with John, Peter said, Look at us. So he gave them his attention, expecting to receive something from them. Then Peter said, Silver and gold I do not have, but what I do have I give you: In the name of Jesus Christ of Nazareth, rise up and walk. And he took him by the right hand and lifted him up, and immediately his feet and ankle bones received strength. So he, leaping up, stood and walked and entered the temple with them— walking, leaping, and praising God... Now as the lame man who was healed held on to Peter and John, all the people ran together to them in the porch which is called Solomon's, greatly amazed. So when Peter saw it, he responded to the people: Men of Israel, why do you marvel at this? Or why look so intently at us, as though by our own power or godliness we had made this man walk?"

Mark 6:1-6 (NKJV): "Then He went out from there and came to His own country, and His disciples followed Him. And when the Sabbath had come, He began to teach in the synagogue. And many hearing Him were astonished, saying, Where did this Man get these things? And what wisdom is this which is given to Him, that such mighty works are performed by His hands! Is this not the carpenter, the Son of Mary, and brother of James, Joses, Judas, and Simon? And are not His sisters here with us? So they were offended at Him. But Jesus said to them, A prophet is not without honor except in his own country, among his own relatives, and in his own house. Now He could do no mighty work there, except that He laid His hands on a few sick people and healed them. And He marveled because of their unbelief. Then He went about the villages in a circuit, teaching."

Mom, I challenge you to read and reread the Scriptures in this letter. In every case, there was no question of Jesus' ability to heal. The most important question that needed to be answered was did the person who needed healing have the faith to be healed.

In several of these scriptures, Jesus said, "according to your faith, be it unto you." He didn't say, "according to my ability" or "according to the power I have now." Jesus had all the power of Heaven at His disposal. The only limitation on that power was the faith of the person who wanted to be healed.

Mom, you have to get this. The power that God used to create the earth, to part the Red Sea, to even raise Jesus from the dead is still available to heal us today. **Romans 8:11 (NKJV)** says that the same Spirit that "raised Christ from the dead will also give life to your mortal bodies through His Spirit who dwells in you."

You could want toast for breakfast, put the bread in the toaster, but if it is unplugged, you will never get toast. The electric current is steadily flowing through the wall with more than enough power to cook the toast, but until you plug in the toaster, you will never have toast.

We plug into the healing power of God by faith, and then healing power flows to us. An excellent example of this principle is the woman with "the issue of blood" in Luke chapter 8. She touched Jesus' garment with faith to be healed, and healing power flowed into her body. Jesus wasn't even aware of what she was doing.

We know that Jesus didn't know who touched Him because He asked, "who touched me?" This seemed odd because Jesus was in a crowd with many touching Him. But Jesus was acknowledging that someone was touching him with a special touch, a touch combined with the faith to be healed. Jesus confirms this by saying "virtue" or power has gone out of me, and then by telling the woman that her faith had made her whole.

The healing power was there inside Jesus but would never have been released unless the woman had the faith and then took accompanying faith steps or actions. Your faith action might be as simple as praying in faith, but healing will not come without faith.

If God just rained down healing on every sick person, there would be no faith required. People who don't know God point to this all the time as proof that God is not good. It sounds like this, "how can God allow all these people to suffer?"

The answer to this question is similar to the question, "why does a good God send people to hell." As Christians, we know that God already sent Jesus as the way to escape hell. Anyone can "call on the Lord and be saved" (Romans 10:13). Salvation requires faith in the Bible truth that Jesus was crucified, died, was buried, and rose on the third day and that His death paid for our sins and that through belief in Him, we have eternal life.

Similarly, escape from the suffering of any sickness or disease requires faith in the Bible truths about healing. Hebrews 11:6 (NKJV) says, "But without faith it is impossible to please Him, for he who comes to God must believe that He is, and that He is a rewarder of those who diligently seek Him." God requires that we believe in Him, that we diligently seek Him in faith, then He "rewards" us with the answer to what we were seeking.

Someone may say that "I know someone who got healed and didn't pray; God just healed them." But we don't know who else may have prayed in faith for that person. God is not trying to keep healing from us; He's trying to get it to us. The only requirement is that we ask in faith. Our faith plugs us into the healing power of God, that is there for all who believe.

How the Word of the Lord Travels

Isaiah 55:11(NKJV): "So shall My word be that goes forth from My mouth; it shall not return to Me void, but it shall accomplish what I please, and it shall prosper in the thing for which I sent it."

Daniel 10:2, 4-6, 12-13 (NKJV): "In those days I, Daniel, was mourning three full weeks… Now on the twenty-fourth day of the first month, as I was by the side of the great river, that is, the Tigris, I lifted my eyes and looked, and behold, a certain man clothed in linen, whose waist was girded with gold of Uphaz! His body was like beryl, his face like the appearance of lightning, his eyes like torches of fire, his arms and feet like burnished bronze in color, and the sound of his words like the voice of a multitude… And he said to me, O Daniel, man greatly beloved, understand the words that I speak to you, and stand upright, for I have now been sent to you. While he was speaking this word to me, I stood trembling. Then he said to me, Do not fear, Daniel, for from the first day that you set your heart to understand, and to humble yourself before your God, your words were heard; and I have come because of your words. But the prince of the kingdom of Persia withstood me twenty-one days; and behold, Michael, one of the chief princes, came to help me, for I had been left alone there with the kings of Persia."

Psalm 103:20-21 (NKJV): "Bless the LORD, you His angels, who excel in strength, who do His word, heeding the voice of His word. Bless the LORD, all you His hosts, you ministers of His, who do His pleasure."

Hebrews 1:13-14 (KJV): "But to which of the angels said he at any time, Sit on my right hand, until I make thine enemies thy footstool? Are they not all ministering spirits, sent forth to minister for them who shall be heirs of salvation?"

Jeremiah 1:12 (KJV): "Then said the LORD unto me, Thou hast well seen: for I will hasten my word to perform it."

Jeremiah 1:12 (NIV): "The LORD said to me, "You have seen correctly, for I am watching to see that my word is fulfilled."

Psalm 107:20 (NKJV) "He sent His word and healed them, and delivered them from their destructions."

Mom, in this letter, I just wanted to share a little bit about the Word of God travels. In Isaiah 55:11, we see God backing up His word with a promise. That promise is that when His Word is released, it won't come back without performing what it is sent to do. The part people miss is how His Word gets sent out in the first place.

God is not just sending out His word to perform things. He did that in the Old Testament in Genesis, where He spoke things into existence. But then, He rested. He now sends His Word out in response to people who pray in faith. A lot of people ask why did God let that happen? Or why didn't God do something?

Since the garden, God has given us authority in the earth. It's like when we grow up and move out of our parent's house. Once we move out, our parents don't just come over uninvited and start doing things in our house. Our parents are often ready to help, but we need to ask for it and invite them in. Pushy or insecure parents might try to force their advice on their kids or keep "popping over" to see if they are still needed. God is not like that. He wants us to invite Him in to help by praying in faith.

Hebrews 11:6 (NKJV) says, "But without faith it is impossible to please Him, for he who comes to God must believe that He is, and that He is a rewarder of those who diligently seek Him." God has set it up that we have to believe that He exists first, then seek Him, reach out to Him in faith, and then He rewards us. He knows all, sees all, and is aware of all our needs, but if He answered our needs without our asking, there would be no faith, no humility, no honoring Him on our part.

When we pray the Word of God, Psalm 103 says that God sends angels in response. These angels that "excel in strength," "do His word," "do His pleasure." Hebrews chapter 1 says that angels are "ministering spirits" sent forth to "minister" to or serve us who are the "heirs of salvation." Now, when I say serve us, I mean that they are indeed doing God's pleasure, which is honoring our prayers of faith with responses.

Daniel is an excellent example of this. Daniel prayed, and an angel showed up. The angel told him that he was sent (by God) in response to Daniel's prayers. The angel also mentioned that Daniel demonstrated humility. Remember that I said praying to God demonstrates faith that He is. It demonstrates faith that He can fix our situation. And praying demonstrates the humility to recognize that He is greater than us; that He is Lord of the Universe.

The angel told Daniel that he was greatly beloved. So are you. The Bible says that God so loved you and me and even the world that He gave His only begotten Son so that if we receive Him as Lord by faith that we would have eternal life. When we pray, God responds out of His love for us. Responding to our prayers of faith gives Him pleasure, and the angels do His pleasure.

In the case of Daniel, we see that angels helped ensure that God's word did not return void. A demon referred to as "the Prince of the kingdom of Persia" tried to stop Daniel's answer. We know it was a demon because he was powerful enough to hinder the first angel and a second, more powerful angel. In fact, a "chief" angel, Michael, had to be called in to help.

In Jer 1:12, we see that God watches over His Word to see that it is fulfilled. What is this word? It's the Word of God that you speak in faith when you pray, believing that He will send a response out of His great love for you.

In at least three places (Matt 24:35, Mark 13:31, Luke 21:33), the Bible says, "heaven and earth shall pass away, but my words shall not pass away." Of course, it's not passing away; Almighty God is watching over His Word and has all the forces and resources of Heaven at His disposal to bring it to pass.

So, from now on, when you pray, I want you to imagine angels flying toward you with answers. I want you to imagine God Himself peeking out over His throne, watching over His Word - the word you prayed in faith - to see that it is fulfilled. All you have to do is wait like Daniel did until the answer comes. I will share with you how to wait in the next letter.

Standing Until The Answer Comes

Hebrews 6:11-12 (NKJV): "And we desire that each one of you show the same diligence to the full assurance of hope until the end, that you do not become sluggish, but imitate those who through faith and patience inherit the promises."

Hebrews 10:35-39 (NIV): "So do not throw away your confidence; it will be richly rewarded. You need to persevere so that when you have done the will of God, you will receive what he has promised. For, in just a little while, he who is coming will come and will not delay...But my righteous one will live by faith. And I take no pleasure in the one who shrinks back. But we do not belong to those who shrink back and are destroyed, but to those who have faith and are saved."

Ephesians 6:13 (NKJV): "Therefore take up the whole armor of God, that you may be able to withstand in the evil day, and having done all, to stand. (having all your armour on... the breastplate and the...and the... and the...etc stand until you see the full manifestation of the promise or until you walk into the gates of heaven."

Daniel 3:17-18 (NKJV) "If that is the case, our God whom we serve is able to deliver us from the burning fiery furnace, and He will deliver us from your hand, O king. But if not, let it be known to you, O king, that we do not serve your gods, nor will we worship the gold image which you have set up."

Oh, Mom, so many people miss it here. They pray scriptures in faith but don't stand until the answer comes. How long will it take? I don't know. Daniel's answer took 21 days. If Daniel had given up, the angel would have had no authority to deliver the answer and take authority over the demon that was trying to prevent the answer from getting there. Abraham and Sarah waited decades.

Dr. Creflo Dollar taught a message that I will never forget called "Faith and Patience the Power Twins." Heb 6:12 says that you have to have both. It's like trying to create a fire with just a match and no wood. Patience is tied to faith. When I pray in faith, I'm not moved if the answer does not come right away.

In Daniel, chapter 3, the "three Hebrew boys" show that kind of faith. They were tied and bound and about to be tossed into the fiery furnace. There was no visible sign that God's deliverance was near. But they did not waiver in their response to the king. They had faith in God's ability to deliver, and that was the end of it.

Abraham acted the same way in response to God's promise for a son in his old age:

Romans 4:17-20 (NIV) As it is written: "I have made you a father of many nations." He is our father in the sight of God, in whom he believed—the God who gives life to the dead and calls into being things that were not. Against all hope, Abraham in hope believed and so became the father of many nations, just as it had been said to him, "So shall your offspring be. Without weakening in his faith, he faced the fact that his body was as good as dead—since he was about a hundred years old—and that Sarah's womb was also dead. Yet he did not waver through unbelief regarding the promise of God, but was strengthened in his faith and gave glory to God."

Let's take a closer look. First was God's promise to Abraham; you will be "the father of many nations." That then became the Word that would not return void, the Word that God was watching over to fulfill. We know that God had the power to call His answer to Abraham's need into existence. God can call things that be not as though they were. He can call you healed, though everyone that knows you knows you're sick. And if you believe Him, your faith in His Word brings the thing that was not into existence: health, healing, victory, deliverance, freedom, etc.

The Bible says Abraham's situation was hopeless, but that Abraham stood up against this hopelessness in faith. The Bible said that Abraham knew that his body (at least his reproductive ability) was as good as dead and that Sarah's was also. He faced the natural facts. But not only did he refuse to give into unbelief, he got strengthened in his faith and was able to give glory to God.

We know that Abraham was 75 when he was told he would have a child (Gen 12:4) and about 100 when the child was born, so about a 25-year wait. During that time, his name changed from Abram to Abraham. So, when Sarah or anyone else called him Abraham, which means father of many nations, he had to respond. He did that for 25 years, waiting in faith!

Now you know that somewhere during that time, Sarah brought Hagar to Abraham as part of a plan to try to fulfill God's plan outside of faith. We know that Hagar had Abraham's child. We also know that God said hey, this isn't my answer. Abraham went on from there, got back on the faith and patience train, and waited to receive God's answer, which was a baby from Abraham and Sarah.

I find it interesting that God didn't hold this momentary lapse, this slip-up, this bit of doubting against Abraham. So much so that God in the Bible calls Abraham the father of faith and that he "did not waver in unbelief." I believe this is like God referring to David as "a man after God's own heart" even after all his mistakes. God looked into David's heart and Abraham's heart and referred to them according to the overall state of their heart and how they finished.

So, Mom, don't be discouraged if you have some days where you feel like you doubted. Just get back on the faith and patience train. God is not watching to catch you if you slip and then judge you. He's watching over His Word to perform it in your life.

Hebrews 10 talks about "not throwing away your confidence" because you know you will be richly rewarded by the God who "rewards those that diligently seek Him" in faith. It talks about "not shrinking" or drawing back away from God's promise even if it takes time. I think you told me, "Every day above ground is a good day." Well, change it to this, "every day above ground is a day that God can still answer your prayer." If you're still on this side, it's not over, no matter how bad it looks!

Ephesians 6:13 says when you have done all to stand in the evil day, keep standing. What's an evil day? An evil day is any day that the devil is attacking your body in sickness and disease or through depression. An evil day is any day where the devil attacks you with doubt and thoughts that God can't heal you. In those "evil" days, the Bible says we have to fight.

We don't fight with earthly weapons, though, but with weapons God provided us. Our "loins girt up with truth"—the belief in the truth of God's Word.

"Feet shod with the gospel of peace and the helmet of salvation"—the good news, the knowledge that we are saved and heirs of God and have a right to receive His promises.

"The breastplate of righteousness"—the knowledge that we are made righteous because of the blood of Jesus, not our own efforts, and that this right standing with God gives us the right to call on Him for deliverance.

"The shield of faith above all things to quench all the fiery darts of the wicked." Faith to quench, to stop, to block everything that the enemy tries to throw at you. These ways include the idea that you won't be healed, that you're going to die, or that you're foolish. It also includes the devil reminding you of others who didn't make it.

"The sword of the spirit." God gave you a way to slice up the devil, to carve him up when he makes the mistake of messing with you. Use the sword of the Spirit to hit him with words backed up by the God of Heaven and his angels.

Finally, in 6:18, it says to "pray with all kinds of prayers (thanksgiving, praise, intercession for others)." Some ways to show your faith are to give thanks for your healing, to praise God for an answer that hasn't even arrived yet, and to be so sure that your answer is coming that you can take time to pray for others!

Mom, this was a lot, but you must have needed it! It poured out of me for you. Read it over and over to encourage yourself. Don't just read the letter. Pull out your Bible, and flip the pages, and read the Scriptures aloud. I learned that from Kenneth Copeland. I don't know why it works better than only reading silently, but it does.

Stand. Persevere. Don't shrink back. Don't throw away your confidence. Don't give up on your faith in God's ability to heal because the answer has taken a long time. Every day above ground is a day for symptoms to diminish, for healing to manifest, and another day to realize that God's truth is more significant than every lie of the devil!

Watch Your Mouth

Mom, have you ever heard somebody say, "watch your mouth"? Like a mom telling her son not to cuss or how to talk around grown folks? There is some spiritual truth related to being careful about what we say.

Genesis 1:3, 9, 27, 2:19 (KJV): "And God said, Let there be light: and there was light…And God said, Let the waters under the heaven be gathered together unto one place, and let the dry land appear: and it was so…So God created man in his own image, in the image of God created he him; male and female created he them…And out of the ground the LORD God formed every beast of the field, and every fowl of the air; and brought them unto Adam to see what he would call them: and whatsoever Adam called every living creature, that was the name thereof."

In these passages from the book of Genesis, we see some important things. We see that God spoke things into existence; whatever He said was so. Then He created us in His image as speaking spirits but in human flesh and blood bodies. As speaking spirits made in His image, the words we say also have creative power. The Bible says whatever Adam said was the name of every living creature, which was its name.

We have heard the scripture from **Proverbs 18:29 (KJV)**, "Death and life are in the power of the tongue: and they that love it shall eat the fruit thereof." But what does it mean? It says that we, as speaking spirits, made in God's image can speak words with creative power, with "fruit," results, or consequences affecting even life and death. We saw Jesus curse a fig tree, and later it withered up and died. But what about human beings?

Proverbs 12:18 (NKJV) says, "There is one who speaks like the piercings of a sword, but the tongue of the wise promotes health." You have heard parents who called their kids stupid or ugly or no good. We may not see the results instantly, but we know that the "fruit" of those words show up later in their children. Something in their kids died, potential, hope, etc.

The same scripture says the tongue of the wise promotes health. Once I learned this, I started to call my daughters beautiful even when they felt they weren't. I learned to speak words of encouragement to them and to my son. You have seen the fruit of that.

The same truths apply to words we speak about our health. We can say oh, I always get the flu in February. We can say I don't think I will get any better or that I will ever be healed. Or we can speak with the "tongue of the wise" and speak words that "promote health." For example, we could say Lord, I thank you that you heard my prayer and I receive the manifestation of my healing"; "Lord, my whole body aches, but I believe that you have heard my prayers and your healing power is at work in my body."

These scriptures from Proverbs are just a small sample of the truth contained in the Bible as it relates to our words:

Proverbs 6:2 (KJV): "Thou art snared with the words of thy mouth, thou art taken with the words of thy mouth."

Proverbs 13:2 (KJV): "A man shall eat good by the fruit of his mouth: but the soul of the transgressors shall eat violence."

Proverbs 13:3 (KJV): "He that keepeth his mouth keepeth his life: but he that openeth wide his lips shall have destruction."

Proverbs 18:7 (KJV): "A fool's mouth is his destruction, and his lips are the snare of his soul."

The Bible uses words like "snared" (caught in a trap), "taken" (captured), "keepeth his life," and destruction" to describe the "fruit" of speaking bad words.

Speaking good words produces good fruit and life in our lives. Speaking good words is also an act of faith. When everything hurts or looks terrible or when every word from the doctor sounds terrible, it takes faith to believe that healing is possible. The Bible says that faith without works is dead/useless (**James 2:20, 26**). Sometimes just speaking what you're believing to happen and thanking God that it is happening is your first step of faith.

> **Matthew 9:28-29 (NKJV)**: "And when He had come into the house, the blind men came to Him. And Jesus said to them, Do you believe that I am able to do this? They said to Him, Yes, Lord. Then He touched their eyes, saying, According to your faith let it be to you."

> **Mark 10:51-52 (NKJV)**: "So Jesus answered and said to him, What do you want Me to do for you? The blind man said to Him, Rabboni, that I may receive my sight. Then Jesus said to him, Go your way; your faith has made you well. And immediately he received his sight and followed Jesus on the road."

In the Scriptures from Matthew 9 and Mark 4, we see Jesus getting the people who wanted healing to speak, to say what they were believing for before it happened. In both cases, Jesus said that the word they spoke was an indication of, evidence of, their faith. After the blind men said, "Yes I believe," Jesus said according to your faith, let it be unto you. He didn't say according to your words, but it meant the same thing because the words spoken were an act of faith. The same was true for the blind man in Mark 10.

In these two separate instances, the words spoken by the blind men, combined with their faith, had the creative power to produce good fruit, in this case, healing. What if the men had said nothing or no I don't believe? I believe that those negative words, words of unbelief, would have resulted in bad fruit, a snare, a loss of an opportunity to receive a miracle.

Revelation 12:11 (NKJV) says, "And they overcame him by the blood of the Lamb and by the word of their testimony, and they did not love their lives to the death." The words of our mouths are so important to overcoming the work of the devil, and his works of sickness and disease. So, watch your mouth!

Whose Plan Was Death?

Hebrews 9:27-28 (NKJV): "And as it is appointed for men to die once, but after this the judgment, so Christ was offered once to bear the sins of many. To those who eagerly wait for Him He will appear a second time, apart from sin, for salvation."

John 10:10 (NKJV): "The thief cometh not, but for to steal, and to kill, and to destroy: I am come that they might have life, and that they might have it more abundantly."

Mom, everybody is going to die. But we forget that was not God's original plan. God's plan, as revealed in Genesis, was that Adam and Eve would live forever in the garden and that they would be "fruitful and multiply" and "replenish the earth." **(Genesis 1:28 KJV)**

Even after the fall, Adam lived to be 930 years old **(Genesis 5:4).** My point was that death was never part of God's original plan for us. He made us in His image and likeness and intended us to live with Him forever. We know that after the fall, He sent Jesus into the earth so that we could have eternal life, even though our physical bodies would die because of Adam's sin.

But when you look back into the account of Adam and Eve in the garden, you see who introduced death into the earth. God told Adam and Eve that if you eat the fruit of the tree of the knowledge of good and evil, you will surely die **(Genesis 2:17).** In Gen 3:4, Satan tells Eve you will not surely die. We know how the story ends. Adam and Eve ate the fruit of the forbidden tree and died instantly. Instantly they became spiritually dead and were put out of the garden to die physically as well.

Following Satan's lie would result in Adam and Eve's spiritual and later physical death. Neither of these deaths was part of God's plan for their lives. We see that not too far after Adam's fall that Satan causes jealousy to rise in Cain's heart and inspires him to murder Abel—the first death by murder. We know the devil inspired this death, from what God told Cain in **Genesis 4:6-8 (NKJV)**:

> "So the LORD said to Cain, "Why are you angry? And why has your countenance fallen? "If you do well, will you not be accepted? And if you do not do well, sin lies at the door. And its desire is for you, but you should rule over it." Now Cain talked with Abel his brother; and it came to pass, when they were in the field, that Cain rose up against Abel his brother and killed him."

My point in sharing all this, mom is to show you that there is one person whose motive is death and murder. John 10:10 is a New Testament scripture that says the devil is a thief that comes to "steal, kill and destroy," but we see it was his way of operating from the beginning. Even before the garden, he tried to steal the glory and the honor that was reserved for God. That's how he ended up cast into the earth in the first place.

In John 10:10, Jesus, the second Adam **(1 Corinthians 15:47 NLT)**, said He came that we might have life and life more abundantly." But this was the same thing the Father, God, had planned for us in the garden. He planned that we would eat from the tree of life and live forever in an abundant life of eternal fellowship with Him.

I shared all this to show without a doubt that God's plan for all of us has always been life. The devil's plan for us has always been to steal from us, to kill us, and to destroy us. So, when you examine life, whatever is in it that is stealing abundant life from you or trying to kill or destroy you is unquestionably from the devil.

In other letters, I will talk to you about the will of God and what the devil can do, but I wanted to lay the foundation for the truth of whose plan the death of man was from the beginning.

How Did They Die?

Mom, I believe the Holy Spirit put it on my heart to go back and investigate how people we have heard of in the Bible died. I believe that part of the selection of names I made was the Holy Ghost, and part of it was random.

What I believed Holy Spirit was trying to show me was that so many of the Old Testament saints just got old and died. I believe the devil, over the years, has gotten people, even our church leaders, to believe that you have to get sick to die or that you have to die of some terrible disease versus just getting old and going home. You don't have to be sick to die. The Bible in **Deuteronomy 34:7** says that Moses died with all "his natural vigor." He was healthy and strong, but just old. Many of the people in these stories reached or passed the age of whatever the Bible was calling old at that the time that they lived.

Today, we say he or she "went home to be with the Lord," but the saying has come to include death by cancer or a tragic accident, or even murder—all of which we blame on God. I pray that as you read these accounts of how and when people died, you will see that often, the great men and women of faith in the Bible just got old and wore out and went home.

If the devil tricks you into believing that some terrible sickness is part of God's plan to take you home, that the God of the universe needs sickness or disease or tragedy to bring you home, then it gives him an open door to sneak into your life and bring these things with him.

Adam old age 930. **Genesis 5:4**

Genesis 25:7-8 (NKJV) This is the sum of the years of Abraham's life which he lived: one hundred and seventy-five years. Then **Abraham** breathed his last and died in a good **old age**, an old man and full of years, and was gathered to his people.

Moses died at the high end of the average lifespan, as described by God at that time. **Genesis 6:3 NLT**: Then the LORD said, "My Spirit will not put up with humans for such a long time, for they are only mortal flesh. In the future, their normal lifespan will be no more than 120 years." **Deuteronomy 34:7 (NKJV)** Moses was one hundred and twenty years old when he died. His eyes were not dim, nor his natural vigor diminished. I like the NLT translation because it says, "normal lifespan" because there are many accounts of people living beyond 120 years old. (Purdom & Menton, 2010)

David: Bible-history.com says that **David** died at age 70:

> "King David died in 960 B.C. at the age of 70, we know he was 70 years old because 1 Kings 2:11 says he reigned for 40 years and 2 Samuel 5:4 says he began his reign at the age of 30. 'David [was] thirty years old when he began to reign, [and] he reigned forty years.' 2 Samuel 5:4 'So David slept with his fathers, and was buried in the city of David. And the days that David reigned over Israel [were] forty years: seven years reigned he in Hebron, and thirty and three years reigned he in Jerusalem.' - 1 Kings 2:10-11"

> (The Tomb of David Monument, n.d.)

Interestingly, at the time of David, the Bible starts referring to people as being old, around the age of 70. Psalm 90:10 says, "The days of our lives are seventy years; and if by reason of strength they are eighty years, yet their boast is only labor and sorrow; for it is soon cut off, and we fly away."

I believe the Bible makes it clear that David likely died of old age. It's humorous to me how the Bible shows that David was nearing death. The Bible paints a clear picture of how David was with beautiful women. So, to determine whether he was about to die, a test was created. They found the most "lovely" woman in the territory and put her in bed with him.

The Bible says he did not "know" her or have sexual relations with her. David's lack of response to the young woman triggered those surrounding David to believe he was about to die. They brought in Nathan, the prophet, and started making sure that David set everything in place for Solomon to succeed him before dying.

"Now King David **was old, advanced in years**; and they put covers on him, but he could not get warm. Therefore his servants said to him, 'Let a young woman, a virgin, be sought for our lord the king, a and let her stand before the king, and let her care for him; and let her lie in your bosom, that our lord the king may be warm.' So they sought for a lovely young woman throughout all the territory of Israel, and found Abishag the Shunammite, and brought her to the king. The young woman was very lovely; and she cared for the king, and served him; but the king did not know her."

I believe that although David only lived to be 70 years old, it was a rough 70 years. Everything we read about David's life as a warrior and fleeing from Saul and his struggles with Absalom wore David out. Though, according to Psalms, he did not die before the age promised in Psalm 90:10.

Rachel: Jacob/Israel's wife Rachel died in childbirth. **Genesis 35 16-18.**

Esther: The Bible doesn't say how she died.

Elijah: Didn't die but met God in the sky in "chariot of fire." **(2 Kings 2:11 NKJV)**

Elisha: Elisha died from sickness or illness. "Now Elisha had been suffering from the illness from which he died. Jehoash king of Israel went down to see him and wept over him. My father! My father! he cried. The chariots and horsemen of Israel!" **(2 Kings 13:14 NIV)**

Sarah: Died of old age. "Sarah lived one hundred and twenty-seven years; these were the years of the life of Sarah. So Sarah died in Kirjath Arba (that is, Hebron) in the land of Canaan, and Abraham came to mourn for Sarah and to weep for her." **(Genesis 23:1-2)**

Mary: (Mother of Jesus): The Bible doesn't say how she died.

Joseph: (Father of Jesus): The Bible doesn't say how he died.

Daniel: The Bible doesn't say how he died, but some theologians estimate that he was at least 82 years old:

> "How did Daniel the prophet die? Answer: The answer to this question is simple. We have no idea how Daniel died. There is no source which is helpful on this at all. However, from Daniel chapter six we know that Daniel survived at least a couple of years into the administration of Persia after Babylon was conquered by Cyrus in 538 BC. We know that Daniel was at least a teenager when he was taken to Babylon in 605 BC (Daniel 1:1). Therefore, Daniel was at least eighty-two years old when the events of Daniel six happened, so he easily Could have died of the normal processes of old age at this point. We do not need to consider any kind of extraordinary means of his death." John Oakes (Oakes, 2017)

Miriam: Did not die of leprosy. Moses prayed for healing/forgiveness. **(Numbers 12:13-14)** Scholars estimate that she was over 125 at the time of her death: "James Ussher estimates her lifespan at 130 years, similar to those of her father Amram (137 years) and Kohath (133 years).” (Ussher, 2016) “Miriam the Prophetess died at the age of 126 (or 127) years. She was the oldest of the three. She died on the tenth day of Nissan, in the year 2487…” (Mindel, n.d.)

Aaron: It appears Aaron’s life was cut short by disobedience: **Numbers 20:23-26, 28 (NKJV):**

> “And the LORD spoke to Moses and Aaron in Mount Hor by the border of the land of Edom, saying: Aaron shall be gathered to his people, for he shall not enter the land which I have given to the children of Israel, because you rebelled against My word at the water of Meribah. Take Aaron and Eleazar his son, and bring them up to Mount Hor; and strip Aaron of his garments and put them on Eleazar his son; for Aaron shall be gathered to his people and die there…Moses stripped Aaron of his garments and put them on Eleazar his son; and Aaron died there on the top of the mountain. Then Moses and Eleazar came down from the mountain.”

Even with his life apparently shortened by disobedience, scholars estimate that he was 123 years old at the time of his death. (Mindel, n.d.)

Joshua: The Bible doesn’t say how he died. “Now it came to pass after these things that Joshua the son of Nun, the servant of the LORD, died, being one hundred and ten years old." **(Joshua 24:29 NKJV)**

Ruth: The Bible does not say how she died, but one theologian estimates that she was at least 90 years. ((The Book of Ruth Timeline, maps, chronology, sermons of Ruth, n.d.)

In every place where the Bible was silent about how a person died, I tried not to guess. The point I was trying to make is that if God were trying to teach us great Bible lessons about how sickness was part of His plan for our death, He would have done so.

The fact that He doesn't is a sign to me that overemphasizing sickness as the primary way that people die is the work of the devil and the work of man. God's original plan was for us to live forever. Words like old, and sick, and dead would have never been in our vocabulary.

I'm releasing my faith to die of old age. Old age for me, and my faith is over 100. I'm not planning to let the devil take me out any sooner through sickness or anything else. I believe I can be like many of these saints. When my work is done and I am old, I can step out of my body and into the presence of God. I believe that you can do the same.

I hope this letter has helped you. I love you, mom!

Do I Deserve to Be Healed?

Romans 5:8 (NKJV): "But God demonstrates his own love for us in this: While we were still sinners, Christ died for us."

1 John 4:10 (NIV): "This is love: not that we loved God, but that he loved us and sent his Son as an atoning sacrifice for our sins."

Hebrews 4:16 (NKJV): "Let us therefore come boldly to the throne of grace, that we may obtain mercy and find grace to help in time of need."

Ephesians 2:8-9 (NKJV): "For by grace you have been saved through faith, and that not of yourselves; it is the gift of God, not of works, lest anyone should boast."

Isaiah 53:5 (NKJV): "But He was wounded for our transgressions, he was bruised for our iniquities;
the chastisement for our peace was upon Him,
and by His stripes we are healed."

1 Peter 2:24 (NKJV): "Who Himself bore our sins
in His own body on the tree, that we, having died to sins,
might live for righteousness—by whose stripes you were healed."

Mom, no one deserves the fantastic gifts that God gives us. He gives us salvation and healing and all His other wonderful blessings out of His great love for us. The Bible tells us that He decided to love us "while we still sinners," even before we loved Him.

While it is true that we don't deserve His amazing gifts, nothing should stop us from receiving them. We start by recognizing that God's grace is what allows us to receive the great gifts that none of us deserve because of any good works we have done (Eph 2:8-9).

Heb 4:16 tells us to "come boldly to the throne of grace, that we may obtain mercy and find grace to help in time of need." It doesn't sound right that we should boldly come to God's throne, asking for something we don't deserve, but that's exactly what God tells us to do.

In my mind, approaching God for grace works like this: I know I don't deserve His grace or His mercy, so it takes the pressure off. I get to have it because He's my daddy, and He said I could have it. He knows everything I have done. Before I was born, He knew what I would do, and He still decided to love me before I got here and to make beautiful gifts like salvation and healing available to me.

Healing is not yours because you deserve it, but because Christ paid for it, along with your sins, on the cross. The Bible in 1Pet 2:24 says, "by whose stripes you were healed." The Greek word *iaomai* is translated "healed" in that passage. It means to cure, to heal, to make whole. A similar verse is found in Isa 53:5, it says by His stripes we are healed." The Hebrew word *rapha* is translated "healed" in that verse, and it means "to heal, make healthful."

The Bible says in **Romans 8:1 (NKJV)** that "There is therefore now no condemnation to those who are in

Christ Jesus, who do not walk according to the flesh, but according to the Spirit." So, if you are feeling condemnation, that is making you think that you are not worthy of God's good gifts, that feeling is not from God.

Constant or recurring condemnation comes from the devil. **Revelation 12:10 (NKJV)** says, "for the accuser of our brethren, who accused them before our God day and night, has been cast down." Day and night, the devil's work is to make us feel condemned. It is one of the ways he steals from us.

If he can't stop us from using our faith to receive our healing, he uses condemnation to make us feel that we don't deserve it. If he succeeds in making us feel condemned, we will give up the healing that Christ made possible. Don't allow that to happen! Come boldly before God's throne of grace and receive the healing that Jesus died for.

Who Are You Listening To?

Proverbs 4:23 (NLT): "Guard your heart above all else, for it determines the course of your life."

The Bible says we should guard our hearts. That means guard what we hear, read, watch, etc. The Bible says in Romans 10 that with the heart, we believe unto salvation. David said, "thy Word I have hid in my heart that I might not sin against you." **(Psalm 119:11)** The heart is a significant place; it's the seat of your beliefs.

One of the dangers to our faith for healing is the words of unbelieving or even well-meaning people who are speaking words contrary to the Bible. If we let their words into our hearts, it can negatively affect our faith.

Mark 5:35-43 (NKJV): "While He was still speaking, some came from the ruler of the synagogue's house who said, Your daughter is dead. Why trouble the Teacher any further? As soon as Jesus heard the word that was spoken, He said to the ruler of the synagogue, Do not be afraid; only believe. And He permitted no one to follow Him except Peter, James, and John the brother of James. Then He came to the house of the ruler of the synagogue, and saw a tumult and those who wept and wailed loudly. When He came in, He said to them, Why make this commotion and weep? The child is not dead, but sleeping. And they ridiculed Him. But when He had put them all outside, He took the father and the mother of the child, and those who were with Him, and entered where the child was lying. Then He took the child by the hand, and said to her, 'Talitha, cumi,' which is translated, 'Little girl, I say to you, arise.' Immediately the girl arose and walked, for she was twelve years of age. And they were overcome with great amazement."

In Mark chapter 5, Jesus in on His way to heal the daughter of the ruler of a synagogue but is delayed while healing the "woman with the issue of blood." Jesus then gets word that the girl is dead. When Jesus gets to the house, He tells the people in the house that the girl is not dead. I believe He did this on purpose to see where their faith was. The people in the house "ridiculed" Him. After Jesus put all the unbelieving people out of the house, he was ready to heal the girl. I also noticed that Jesus only allowed three of the disciples to accompany Him. Peter, James, and John are often referred to as Jesus' "inner circle."

Jesus' example is a good one for us to follow. If we are facing a dangerous, perhaps even life-threatening situation, we can't have anybody around us saying things that take away or that detract from our faith. That is not the time to hear negative words, words that go against the truth of the Word of God.

The Traditions of Men

2 Timoth 3:16 (NKJV): "All Scripture is given by inspiration of God, and is profitable for doctrine, for reproof, for correction, for instruction in righteousness."

2 Peter 1:16 (NKJV): "For we did not follow cunningly devised fables when we made known to you the power and coming of our Lord Jesus Christ, but were eyewitnesses of His majesty."

1 Corinthians 2:4-5 (NKJV): "And my word and my preaching, not in persuasive words of wisdom, but in demonstration of the Spirit and of power; that your faith might not stand in men's wisdom, but in God's power."

2 Peter 1:20-21 (NLT): "Above all, you must realize that no prophecy in Scripture ever came from the prophet's own understanding, or from human initiative. No, those prophets were moved by the Holy Spirit, and they spoke from God."

2 Timothy 2:15 (NKJV): "Be diligent to present yourself approved to God, a worker who does not need to be ashamed, rightly dividing the word of truth."

Mark 7:13 (NKJV): "Making the word of God of no effect through your tradition which you have handed down. And many such things you do."

1 Corinthians 1:17 (NKV): "For Christ did not send me to baptize, but to preach the gospel, not with wisdom of words, lest the cross of Christ should be made of no effect."

Mom, as Christians, we are supposed to believe that the Bible is the Word of God. 2 Tim 3:16 says that we are supposed to use the Bible to build our doctrine and our beliefs on. For us, the Bible is not filled with "fables," man-made stories, or words that came from the understanding of a man. We believe that the Holy Ghost inspired men to write what they wrote, or they were "eyewitnesses" **(2 Peter 1:16)** of the works of Christ.

2 Timothy 2:15 encourages us to study the Word of God so that we can rightly "divide" or apply it. This is so important because, just as the Bible can be rightly interpreted, it can be wrongly interpreted.

I have heard so many wrong interpretations of the Bible regarding healing. That's not the worst part. The worst part is that I have heard so much preached about healing that's not even in the Bible. The things I have heard come from men's ideas or religious traditions.

Jesus said that we could make the Word of God of "no effect," no power, because of our traditions. Religious tradition can get into our hearts and make of "no effect" the Word of God that is hidden there.

One biblical example was Jesus healing a man on the Sabbath. The religious tradition said that no work could be done on the Sabbath, and if Jesus had followed that tradition, the man would not have been healed that day.

A more recent tradition I have seen is the placement of one chair at the altar during an altar call. After that, the words, "Would there be one, would there be one?" are said. The church believes for a great end-time harvest, but the one-chair-would-there-be-one tradition hinders the manifestation.

Here are some sayings I have heard that make the Word of God of no effect in healing. They are: "Lord, if it be thy will to heal me," "God plucked a flower out of His garden," "She had an early graduation to Heaven," "God needed him in Heaven," and "She was healed in death."

Nowhere in Scripture do we see Jesus tell someone that it was not His will or the Father's will to heal them. Nowhere do you see God ending someone's life early because He needed them in Heaven. When God took Elijah and Enoch to Heaven early, He took them alive. God has the angels in Heaven. He doesn't need us to do anything. There is nowhere in Scripture where you can find an example to support that tradition.

God has been around for countless multiplied trillions of years times infinity. There is a phrase that says 1,000 years for us is really like one day with God. Since God is and has always been, this saying is not too far off. Therefore, there is no need for Him to take us early because, from His perspective, we are only on the earth for a short time.

Traditions like these don't make any sense, and they have no Scriptural support. Further, they are dangerous. What's the danger? Hearing them over and over can cause them to settle into our hearts and weaken our faith. These traditions make the Word of God of "none effect" and can prevent us from being healed.

If you believe that God is going to take you home early, why would you use your faith to resist sickness and death? If you believe that it's not God's will to heal you, despite all the examples in the Bible, you might not persevere in faith until you receive the manifestation of your healing.

Again, I treat these traditions as dangerous and with high potential for harm. Those are powerful words, but I stand by them because these traditions can be life-threatening. I never forget Gloria Copeland asking, do you believe that is the will of God to "let cancer eat the life out of your body? God doesn't need sickness' help to bring you home."

These traditions are what the Bible calls "the persuasive words of wisdom" and "men's wisdom." Men created these traditions because they could not explain why some people did not get healed. **1 Corinthians 13:12 (NKJV)** says, "For now we see through a glass, darkly; but then face to face: now I know in part; but then shall I know even as also I am known."

It is true that we don't know everything, and sometimes we can't say for sure why someone did not get healed. However, we should just admit that we don't know rather than make up a tradition that slanders the character of the Father, denies His power, and tries to diminish the greatness of His love for us.

Jesus said I only speak what I hear the Father say. If Jesus, as the Son of God, only spoke or repeated what the Father said, no pastor, elder, deacon, bishop, apostle, prophet, missionary, man or woman of God should take the liberty to go outside the Word of the Father, the Word of God.

If one of our leaders doesn't know the scriptural answer, they should say they don't know versus responding in their own wisdom or tradition.

Only the words of God are promised to happen. As eloquent or enticing as a man or woman's words are, they should never be trusted over the Word of God. Why? Because they don't have the power to back them up.

Any words that directly contradict the written Word of God should be quickly and lovingly rejected.

The Thorn in the Flesh

Mom, I'm praying to write on this subject as simply as I can. Theologians have written entire books on this subject. I especially pray for the Holy Spirit's guidance on this because so many people have been tripped up on "the thorn in the flesh as it pertains to healing." I believe the devil has used a misunderstanding of this Scriptural account to steal healings from people by getting them to believe that their sickness is their thorn.

First, Paul is the only person in Scripture referred to as having a thorn in the flesh. When it comes to healing, there are so many examples of how Jesus healed multitudes of people. But the devil wants you to focus on the one who appears not to have received his healing. The truth is the Bible never says that Paul was sick.

In **2 Corinthians 12:7,** Paul says that he got this "thorn" because of the abundance of his revelations. The revelations that Paul received were so many and so powerful that they fill most of the New Testament. No person recorded in the New Testament received more revelation than Paul, so that is likely why he is the only person recorded to have ever received a "thorn."

This is important because none of us have ever received that amount of revelation from God, but we want to be quick to say that we would get a "thorn" in the flesh, which is the reason Paul said he got it.

Where did Paul get the "thorn" from? The Bible says it was "the messenger of Satan," but nearly everyone who talks about Paul's thorn in the flesh makes it seem like God gave it to him.

Years ago, I learned from Gloria Copeland that this "thorn" was a demon sent by the devil to keep Paul from spreading his revelations.

The Greek word for messenger used in this Scripture is "aggelos." It refers to an actual messenger, a sent one. (BlueLetterBible, n.d.) Another meaning is "angel." So, if you reread the passage, it would read, "There was given to me the angel of Satan to buffet me."

Mom, to me, this has always made the most sense. I believe this demon stirred up the crowd everywhere Paul went to preach and resulted in him being stoned and jailed, and harassed everywhere he went.

I believe this demon also had a hand in the three shipwrecks Paul suffered. I have studied this out and will put some additional Scriptural references of what I am describing at the end of this letter.

I don't believe Paul was sick because of all the things he overcame while he was preaching **2 Corinthians 11:23-27 (NKJV):**

"Are they ministers of Christ?—I speak as a fool—
I am more: in labors more abundant, in stripes
above measure, in prisons more frequently, in
deaths often. From the Jews five times I received
forty stripes minus one. Three times I was beaten
with rods; once I was stoned; three times I was
shipwrecked; a night and a day I have been in the
deep; in journeys often, in perils of waters, in perils
of robbers, in perils of my own countrymen, in
perils of the Gentiles, in perils in the city, in perils in
the wilderness, in perils in the sea, in perils among
false brethren; in weariness and toil, in
sleeplessness often, in hunger and thirst, in fastings
often, in cold and nakedness—"

I don't believe that someone with any debilitating
disease could have kept traveling and preaching under
these circumstances. In Acts chapter 14, the Jews at
Antioch stoned Paul so severely that he seemed dead. He
apparently didn't even show any signs of life while they
drug him out of the city, or they would have finished him
off.

Acts 14:19-20 (NKJV): "Then Jews from Antioch
and Iconium came there; and having persuaded the
multitudes, they stoned Paul and dragged him out
of the city, supposing him to be dead. However,
when the disciples gathered around him, he rose
up and went into the city. And the next day he
departed with Barnabas to Derbe."

How does a person look who has been stoned to death? I always imagine massive head trauma, broken bones, massive bleeding. It's hard to believe Paul had a life-threatening or terminal illness on top of all he suffered, especially when the Bible doesn't mention it, and Paul doesn't say anything about it in his list of the perils he faced.

I believe the angel/messenger of Satan interpretation makes the most sense when you consider God's response. Paul asked three times for the "thorn" to be removed. But because the "thorn" was a demon, God said, "My grace is sufficient for thee **(2 Corinthians 12:9 KJV)**.

We can pray until we turn blue, and God is not going to take the devil away. The devil has an appointed time to be taken away, as described in the book of Revelations. Until then, God gives us the grace to overcome everything that the devil throws at us.

The thorn in the flesh is an expression that could easily be interpreted as a thorn in my side:

"**thorn** in your **side**. Someone or something that continually causes problems for you: Money problems have been a **thorn** in your **side** since the day we got married. Health Inspectors are a **thorn** in the **side** of most restaurants.

(Dictionary, n.d.)

I believe the devil assigned a demon to be a thorn in Paul's side wherever he went. Even though the demon assigned to Paul stirred up violent trouble and likely shipwrecks, he couldn't keep Paul from being exalted and spreading the revelations that he received from God.

Some people read 2 Cor 12:7 and say that God was the one trying to keep Paul humble because of the great revelations Paul was given. That's not the character of a good God, to give a good gift and then punish you with a thorn for receiving it.

No, it's the character of the devil to steal, kill, and destroy. We know the devil stirred up the crowd through the chief priest and the elders to choose Barabbas over Jesus even though King Herod did not want to crucify Him. **(Matthew 27:15-21)**

The devil threw everything at Paul and couldn't kill him because of the grace of God on Paul's life. We know that Paul didn't die until he was ready.

Philippians 1:21-25 (NKJV): "For to me, to live is Christ, and to die is gain. But if I live on in the flesh, this will mean fruit from my labor; yet what I shall <u>choose</u> I cannot tell. For I am hard-pressed between the two, having a desire to depart and be with Christ, which is far better. Nevertheless to remain in the flesh is more needful for you. And being confident of this, I know that I shall remain and continue with you all for your progress and joy of faith."

Jesus said no man take my life; I lay it down **(John 10:17-18)**. I believe the same grace was on Paul. Paul said that he "chose" to live, to "remain and continue" his work versus die. He did not die until after he had finished his work: "I have fought the good fight, I have finished the race, I have kept the faith." **(2 Timothy 4:7 NKJV)**

The thorn in the flesh thinking is a trick of the devil to keep you from fighting a sickness because you think it is God's will for you to keep it. Nowhere in the Bible does Jesus tell someone who asks for healing that it's their "thorn in the flesh" and that He will give them the grace to keep suffering from that sickness.

Mom, that may have been a lot to understand, but the essential things to remember are that Paul is the only one the Bible says ever had a thorn, and neither the Bible nor Paul said the thorn was a sickness. Also, since Paul got the thorn because of the abundance of his revelations, most of us don't have to ever worry about getting a thorn in the flesh.

Multitudes/crowds/mobs stirred up against Paul: (Acts 13:45-50, Acts 14:2, Acts 14:19, Acts 17:5, Acts 17:13, Acts 21:27-32).

Close the Door!

Ephesians 4:27 (KJV): "Neither give place to the devil."

Job 1:10 (KJV): "Hast not thou made an hedge about him, and about his house, and about all that he hath on every side? thou hast blessed the work of his hands, and his substance is increased in the land."

Ecclesiastes 10:8 (KJV): "He that diggeth a pit shall fall into it; and whoso breaketh an hedge, a serpent shall bite him."

Ezekiel 22:30 (KJV): "And I sought for a man among them, that should make up the hedge, and stand in the gap before me for the land, that I should not destroy it: but I found none."

The word "hedge: used in the Old Testament Scriptures above means fence or wall. In Job chapter one, the devil complains about a fence or a wall that God has put around Job and all that he has. In Eze 22:30, God said that He was looking for a man to stand in prayerful intercession and build a wall of prayer.

I believe that we have an invisible wall or fence of protection around us. I believe it's made up of angels that are like spiritual bodyguards that go around protecting us from danger and the traps of the enemy.

The terrible thing about every fence is that the gate can be left open, and then the fence is useless for keeping things out. Eph 4:27 says, "neither give place to the devil."

You may be thinking, who would give place to the devil? Well, there are a lot of ways we can give place to the devil. One of them is disobedience.

The most significant example of this is in the Garden of Eden. Adam and Eve's disobedience allowed the devil to come in and take the authority God had given man on the earth, and it also led to their spiritual and later physical death.

In Gen 4:7 (NKJV), God told Cain, "sin lies at the door. And its desire is for you." We know that Cain didn't listen, and through jealousy and anger, opened a door that led to the murder of Abel.

We can open the door to sickness by how we treat our bodies. Our bodies are a gift from God, and He expects us to take care of them and not abuse them. We can abuse them by overeating, abusing alcohol or drugs, smoking, not getting proper rest, ignoring the doctor's instructions, overwork, sexual promiscuity, and any other number of ways. When we abuse our bodies, we open the door to disease, injury, and death.

One of my old Pastors, Dwayne Freeman, said, "At funerals, we need to stop saying, 'God took him.' We need to say, 'the cigarettes took him' or 'that alcohol took him.'" What he said makes sense. People open the door to the devil by abusing their bodies, and the devil brings cancer or liver damage, and then they say, why did God allow this to happen to me? Or if they die, their loved ones say why did God take him so soon?

I remember praying for a man in my office in the early 1990s. Everybody believed he would pull through. The Holy Spirit, however, showed me that his intense bitterness and hatred of his ex-wife was the source of his sickness and that unless he repented of it, he would die. I was, as were many coworkers, aware of the feelings he had towards his ex-wife. He displayed great passion and anger when the subject of his ex-wife came up. When he died, it was puzzling to most, but I remembered what the Holy Spirit revealed to me.

Mom, I do not believe in relying on stories and personal experiences. All doctrine worth standing on must have its foundation in the Word of God. Our personal experience and the stories of others can reinforce or confirm the Bible, but we can't let our faith rest on personal experience alone.

Hebrews 12:15 (KJV): "Looking diligently lest any man fail of the grace of God; lest any root of bitterness springing up trouble you, and thereby many be defiled."

In Heb 12:15, the Greek word "miaino" is translated defiled. (BlueLetterBible, n.d.) It means to stain, pollute, contaminate, defile with sins. The English word "fail" in the phrase "fail the grace of God" comes from the Greek word "hystereō." (BlueLetterBible, n.d.) It means: "to be left behind in the race and so fail to reach the goal, to fall short of the end, fail to become a partaker, to be in want of, lack." (BlueLetterBible, n.d.)

Wow. Mom, that means that if I hold onto bitterness in my heart, it causes me trouble, stains my heart, and defiles it with sin. More importantly, that sin may cause me to miss and fall short of the grace of God that I need to deal with that sin. This falling short is an open door to Satan that allows him to come in and cause us trouble, to steal, kill, and destroy in our lives.

> **Acts 8:22-24 (Berean Study Bible)**: "Repent, therefore, of your wickedness, and pray to the Lord. Perhaps He will forgive you for the intent of your heart. For I see that you are poisoned by bitterness and captive to iniquity. Then Simon answered, Pray to the Lord for me, so that nothing you have said may happen to me."

(Biblehub.com, n.d.)

In Acts 8:23, we see that bitterness is equated to poison and tied to sin's captivity. We can't afford to keep bitterness in our heart and leave the door open to Satan. We must repent of bitterness just as Simon the sorcerer did so that nothing that devil has planned for us will happen.

Medical science has also discovered the truth of the Bible as it relates to bitterness, anger, unforgiveness, and our health:

> "Whether it's a simple spat with your spouse or long-held resentment toward a family member or friend, unresolved conflict can go deeper than you

may realize—it may be affecting your physical health. The good news: Studies have found that the act of forgiveness can reap huge rewards for your health, lowering the risk of heart attack; improving cholesterol levels and sleep; and reducing pain, blood pressure, and levels of anxiety, depression and stress. And research points to an increase in the forgiveness-health connection as you age.

There is an enormous physical burden to being hurt and disappointed," says Karen Swartz, M.D., director of the Mood Disorders Adult Consultation Clinic at The Johns Hopkins Hospital. Chronic anger puts you into a fight-or-flight mode, which results in numerous changes in heart rate, blood pressure and immune response. Those changes, then, increase the risk of depression, heart disease and diabetes, among other conditions. Forgiveness, however, calms stress levels, leading to improved health." (Karen Swartz, n.d.)

"Chronic and intense anger has been linked with Coronary Heart Disease, stroke, cancer and common physical illnesses including colds and flu, and generally poorer health; as well as increased risk-taking, poor decision-making and substance misuse… "Anger has also been linked with mental health problems including depression and self-harm." (Kirkpatrick, n.d.)

"And studies suggest bitterness, and the feelings of anger and depression that accompany it, may be linked to health issues like cardiovascular problems and a weak immune system." (Koerner, 2012)

Mom, the last open door that I want to talk about may be the most important. The door that I am talking about is the door to fear. **2 Timothy 1:7 (NKJV)** says, "For God has not given us a spirit of fear, but of power and of love and of a sound mind."

The reason closing the door to fear is so important is that fear flips everything in that Scripture around. It steals our soundness of mind and makes us worried and anxious. It robs us of our power and confidence as we try to stand boldly against sickness and even death. Finally, it makes us doubt the love of God for us and question whether He is helping us as we believe for healing.

Jesus cautioned Jairus not to be afraid in **Mark 5:35-43 (NKJV)**: "While He was still speaking, some came from the ruler of the synagogue's house who said, 'Your daughter is dead. Why trouble the Teacher any further?' As soon as Jesus heard the word that was spoken, He said to the ruler of the synagogue, 'Do not be afraid; only believe.'"

Jesus knew that one of the greatest enemies of healing was fear, so He helped Jairus confront that fear first before going to heal his daughter. Later in that story, we find that Jairus' home was filled with people that did not believe that his daughter could be healed. In fact, they ridiculed Jesus.

Jesus kicked them all out, but it's easy to see how they could have fueled Jairus' fear if Jesus had not dealt with it beforehand. The faith of Jairus and his wife was key to their daughter's recovery. Fear in Jairus' heart could have spread to his wife and stolen the miracle of their daughter's recovery.

One of the best books I have found about the open door of fear is "Uprooting the Spirit of Fear" by Dr. Creflo A. Dollar. I want to share some of his wisdom here:

> "Fear gives place to the devil, thus allowing him to operate freely. That was precisely what took place with the disciples in the storm-tossed boat. Their fear in the beginning stages of the storm gave Satan room to really start tearing things up.
>
> Fear allowed the storm to get to a point where it might have destroyed them. That is why Jesus exclaimed, "where is your faith?" when He woke up...
>
> There's no way for Satan to operate destructively in your life unless you give place to him. You may ask how do you give place to the devil? You give place to the devil by paying attention to his words and thereby beginning to operate in fear...

Unchecked and unreversed, fear will open the door for the devil to come in kill steal and destroy...your fear has given place to the devil to do his destructive work.

Fear comes by hearing, and hearing means "by words" ...Fear may come through the devil's words directly into your mind or it may enter through the words of other people. For example, fear may enter through your paying attention not only to a doctor but to a friend or relative speaking negatively... Guard the "gates" of your soul. Your eyes and ears are gateways to your mind and spirit...

For the thing which I greatly feared is come upon me, and that which I was afraid of is come unto me. Job 3:25 Job's fear caused God's hedge of protection around him to be lifted. God did not lift the Hedge; Job's fear did." (Dollar, 1994)

The Bible says, "Out of the abundance of the heart, the mouth speaks" **(Luke 6:45)**. If fear is in your heart, fear-filled words will come out of your mouth. If you hear yourself saying words of fear and doubt coming out of your mouth, just repent and close the door.

Fear magnifies the sickness and tries to make it more powerful than the Word of God. Through fear, the devil tries to make it seem like your illness, and your condition are too bad for the Word of God to work on it.

My pastor, Dr. Michael Maiden, said, "pray the answer (from Scripture) don't pray the problem. Prayer is not informing God about the problem; it's praying the answer to the situation from the Word of God."

Fear gets you talking more about the problem and how big it is instead of how big our God is and how powerful His Word is.

Close the door to fear today! And keep it closed!

Healing Checklist

[ ] Expect to receive what you prayed for (Mark 11:24)
[ ] Thank God in advance for your healing
[ ] Repent of all unbelief and words spoken contrary to your healing (Mark 9:24, Hebrews 4:16)
[ ] Stop sinning against your body/close any open doors (overeating, eating foods that are bad for you, smoking, alcohol in excess, poor exercise habits, etc.)
[ ] Receive the mercy and grace of God (Hebrews 4:16)
[ ] Repent of all unforgiveness, bitterness
[ ] Have Elders lay hands on you, anoint with oil, pray (James 5:14-15)
[ ] Take prescribed medicine
[ ] Follow the doctor's orders/advice
[ ] Prayer of faith by others (James 5:15)
[ ] Laying on of hands (Mark 16:18, Acts 28:8)
[ ] Bind and loose (Bind sickness and spirits causing sickness/disease and loose God's healing power, the "quickening" of the Holy Spirit (Matthew 18:18, Romans 8:11)
[ ] Repent if you have taken communion "unworthily" (1 Corinthians 11:27-30)
[ ] Fasting (yourself, others on your behalf) (Isaiah 58:8, Mark 9:29)
[ ] Find one or two more and pray in "agreement" for your healing (Matthew 18:19)
[ ] Confess that you are spiritually covered by the "Blood of Jesus"; that it stands between you and Satan's power to keep you sick. (Revelation 12:11 (NKJV) "And they overcame him by the blood of the Lamb... word of their testimony.)
[ ] Find healing Scriptures to confess in faith over your life. Pray answers (from Scripture); don't pray the problem.

[ ] Remind yourself that Jesus is on your side (Romans 8:34, 1 John 3:8)

*Mom, this is just a checklist of everything I could think of that people have used to be healed. I didn't write letters on each topic, but I included Scriptures. If healing is not manifesting in your body, prayerfully review this list.

A Relationship With God

1. **God loves you very dearly and has an amazing purpose and plan for your life.**

We love Him because He first loved us. I John 4:19

For God so loved the world that He gave His only begotten Son, that whoever believes in Him should not perish but have everlasting life. John 3:16

The thief does not come except to steal, and to kill, and to destroy. I have come that they may have life, and that they may have it more abundantly. John 10:10

2. **Because of sin, man is separated from God and cannot know and experience His love and purposes.**

For all have sinned and fall short of the glory of God. Romans 3:23

For the wages of sin is death, but the gift of God is eternal life in Christ Jesus our Lord. Romans 6:23.

3. **Jesus Christ came to earth and died on the cross for our sins. He rose from the dead and is the only way to a relationship with God. Through Jesus, we can know God's love and purpose for our life.**

But God demonstrates His own love toward us, in that while we were still sinnners, Christ died for us. Romans 5:8

Jesus said to him, "I am the way, the truth, and the life. No one comes to the Father except through Me. John 14:6

4. **Jesus invites us to open up to God and have an intimate relationship with Him.**

Behold, I stand at the door and knock. If anyone hears My voice and opens the door, I will come in to him and dine with him, and he with Me. Revelation 3:20

5. **Our responsibility is to believe and receive Jesus Christ as our Saviour and Lord.**

But as many as received Him, to them He gave the right to become children of God, to those who believe in His name. John 1:12

6. **When we receive Christ, we do so by faith, believing in what He did on the cross, not in our own ability or works.**

For by grace you have been saved through faith, and that not of yourselves; it is the gift of God, not of works, lest anyone should boast. Ephesians 2:8-9

7. **You can receive Christ now by faith and enter into a new relationship with God through prayer.**

If you confess with your mouth the Lord Jesus and believe in your heart that God has raised Him from the dead, you will be saved. For with the heart one believes unto righteousness, and with the mouth confession is made unto salvation. For the Scripture says, "Whosoever believes on Him will not be put to shame." For there is no distinction between Jew and Greek, for the same Lord over all is rich to all who call upon Him. For "whoever calls on the name of the Lord shall be saved." Romans 10:9-13

Here is a suggested prayer:

Father I come to You in the name of Jesus Christ and I thank you for sending Your Son to die for me. Jesus, I recognize my need for You. I thank You for dying on the cross for my sins, and I open my heart to You right now. I receive your forgiveness for my sins and I thank You for giving me eternal life. I receive you ad my Saviour and Lord. I invite You to come in and be the Lord of my life. Show me Your love and lead me to become the person You want me to be. I receive the Father's love and my adoption as Father God's child.

If this prayer echoes the desire of your heart, I invite you to pray it right now and Jesus will come into your life, as He promised.

*This segment comes from the book "God Loves Me and I Love Myself Overcoming the Resistance to Loving Yourself," written by Mark DeJesus Copyright 2016 Mark DeJesus & Turning Hearts Ministries
www.markdejesus.com

(DeJesus, 2016)

Other Books By the Author:

Amazon
https://rebrand.ly/Ivan-Thompson-Amazon

Audible
https://rebrand.ly/Ivan-Thompson-Audible

Here is a list of the e-book & print titles that I have available on Amazon:

- *** 25 Essential Bible Verses for Christian Business Leaders**
- **25 Versículos Esenciales de la Biblia Para Líderes de Negocios Cristianos**
- ***25 Bible Verses for Dads**
- **25 Versículos Bíblicos para Papás: Un Diario de Reflexión**
- ***A Tsunami of Sadness**
- **Un Tsunami de Tristeza**
- ***Hope Deferred Overcoming Discouragement and Faltering Hope**
- **Esperanza Frustrada: Superando el Desánimo y la Falta de Esperanza**
- **Finding Next A Book of Divine Seasons**
- **Financial Testimonies Stories of God's Grace and Provision**
- **Financial Testimonies II**
- ***First Responders a Revelation of the Love of Jesus**

- **Primeros en Responder: "Una Revelación del Amor de Jesús" (Spanish Edition)**
- Increasing Your Skills and Abilities in Any Area
- Letters to Build a Young Man's Confidence
- *Lifesaving The Importance of Hearing the Voice of God
- PODRÍA SALVAR TU VIDA: La importancia de escuchar la voz de Dios
- *Lifesaving Volume II Hardening Your Heart to the Voice of God
- Podría Salvar Tu Vida Volumen II : Endurecer el Corazón a la Voz de Dios
- *The Bible Promises of Healing 16 Letters for Mom
- **Promesas de Curación de la Biblia : 16 Cartas para Mamá**
- The Making of a Great America Where the Founding Fathers and the Church Fell Short
- The Making of a Great America Uprooting the Spirit of Racism
- The Making of a Great America Made in the Image of Trump
- *You Should Detours and Distractions to Divine Destiny
- Usted Debería: Distracciones Y Desvíos Del Destino Divino
- Fit @ 50
- No Grandma It's an e-book
- The Air Force's Black Ceiling
- The Air Force's Black Pilot Training Experience
- The Air Force's Black Pilot State of the Union

***Also available in Spanish**

Here is a list of the audiobook titles that I have available on Audible:

- **The Making of a Great America: Where the Founding Fathers and the Church Fell Short**
- The Making of a Great America: Made in Trump's Image
- **A Tsunami of Sadness**
- **Financial Testimonies: Stories of God's Favor, Grace, and Provision**
- **25 Essential Bible Verses for Christian Business Leaders**
- **25 Versículos Esenciales de la Biblia para Líderes de Negocios Cristianos**
- **You Should Distractions & Detours to Divine Destiny**
- **Usted Debería: Distracciones Y Desvíos Del Destino Divino**
- **The Bible Promises of Healing 16 Letters for Mom**
- **First Responders a Revelation of the Love of Jesus**
- **25 Essential Bible Verses for Dads**
- **Increasing Your Skills and Abilities in Any Area**
- **Letters to Build a Young Man's Confidence**
- **No Grandma It's an e-Book!**
- **The Air Force's Black Ceiling**

Bibliography

Biblehub.com. (n.d.). *Acts 8:23*. Retrieved from Biblehub.com:
        http://biblehub.com/acts/8-23.htm

BlueLetterBible. (n.d.). Retrieved from BlueLetterBible.org:
        https://www.blueletterbible.org/nkjv/heb/12/15/p0/t_
        conc_1145015

DeJesus, M. (2016). God Loves Me and I Love Myself
        Overcoming the Resistance to Loving Yourself. Mark
        DeJesus and Turning Hearts Ministries.

Dictionary, C. (n.d.). *Definition of thorn in your side*. Retrieved
        from dictionary.cambridge.org:
        https://dictionary.cambridge.org/us/dictionary/english/
        thorn-in-your-side

Dollar, C. (1994). Uprooting the Spirit of Fear. In D. C. Dollar,
        Uprooting the Spirit of Fear (pp. 14-15, 35-36). Tulsa
        Oklahoma: Harrison House.

Karen Swartz, M. (n.d.). *Healthy Aging: Forgiveness: Your Health
        Depends on It*. Retrieved from Hopkinsmedicine.org:
        https://www.hopkinsmedicine.org/health/healthy_agin
        g/healthy_connections/forgiveness-your-health-
        depends-on-it

Kirkpatrick, T. (n.d.). *What Does the Bible Say About Anger?*
        Retrieved from lifehopeandtruth.com:
        https://lifehopeandtruth.com/change/sin/what-does-
        the-bible-say-about-anger/

Koerner, K. (2012, Feb 6). *Can Being Bitter Make You Sick?*
        Retrieved from greatist.com:
        https://greatist.com/happiness/can-being-bitter-make-
        you-sick

Mindel, N. (n.d.). *Aaron and Miriam*. Retrieved from
Chabad.org:
http://www.chabad.org/library/article_cdo/aid/112070
/jewish/Aaron-and-Miriam.htm

Oakes, J. (2017, Jan 11). *How Did Daniel Die*. Retrieved from
evidenceforchistianity.org:
http://evidenceforchristianity.org/how-did-daniel-die/

Purdom, D. G., & Menton, D. D. (2010, May 27). *Did Adam and
Noah Really Live Over 900 Years of Age*. Retrieved from
answersingenesis.org:
https://answersingenesis.org/bible-
timeline/genealogy/did-adam-and-noah-really-live-
over-900-years/

The Book of Ruth Timeline, maps, chronology, sermons of Ruth.
(n.d.). Retrieved from www.bible.ca:
http://www.bible.ca/archeology/bible-archeology-
timeline-date-chronology-of-ruth-1300bc.htm

The Tomb of David Monument. (n.d.). Retrieved from
www.bible-history.com: http://www.bible-
history.com/sketches/ancient/tomb-david.html

Ussher, J. (2016, Jul 12). *Miriam*. Retrieved from
conservapedia.com:
http://www.conservapedia.com/Miriam

Winnail, D. S. (2002, July). *DEFEATING DISEASE: HOW THE BIBLE
CAN HELP*. Retrieved from Tomorrowsworld.org:
https://www.tomorrowsworld.org/magazines/2002/jul
y-august/defeating-disease-how-the-bible-can-help

Scripture quotations marked (KJV) are taken from the King
James Version of the Bible. Those marked (NKJV) are taken

from the New King James Version. Those marked (NIV) are taken from the New International Version. Those marked (NLT) are from the New Living Translation. Those marked (ASV) are from the American Standard Version. Those marked (ESV) are from the English Standard Version. Those marked (WEB) are from the Webster's version of the Bible. Most of the scriptures cited come from www.BlueLetterBible.org